The Magic of Spinach

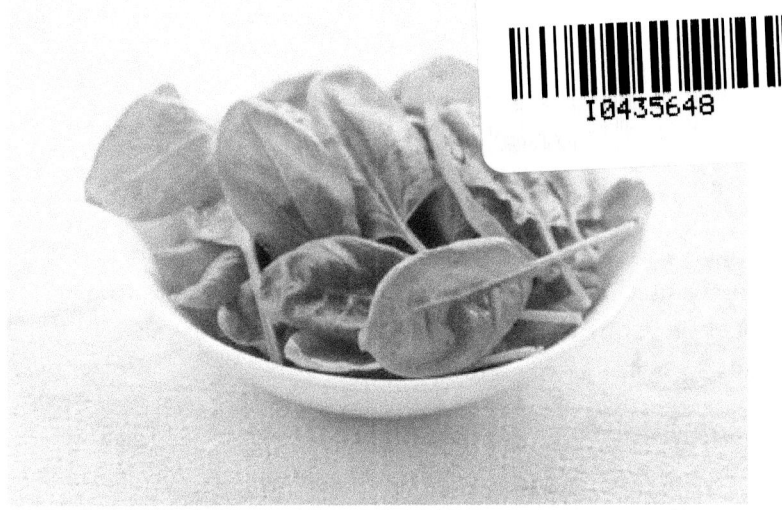

I0435648

Dueep J. Singh

Health Learning Series

Mendon Cottage Books

JD-Biz Publishing

Disclaimer

The information is this book is provided for informational purposes only. It is not intended to be used and medical advice or a substitute for proper medical treatment by a qualified health care provider. The information is believed to be accurate as presented based on research by the author.

The contents have not been evaluated by the U.S. Food and Drug Administration or any other Government or Health Organization and the contents in this book are not to be used to treat cure or prevent disease.

The author or publisher is not responsible for the use or safety of any diet, procedure or treatment mentioned in this book. The author or publisher is not responsible for errors or omissions that may exist.

Warning

The Book is for informational purposes only and before taking on any diet, treatment or medical procedure, it is recommended to consult with your primary health care provider.

Check out some of the other Healthy Gardening Series books at Amazon.com

Gardening Series on Amazon

Check out some of the other Health Learning Series books at Amazon.com

Health Learning Series on Amazon

Table of Contents

Introduction

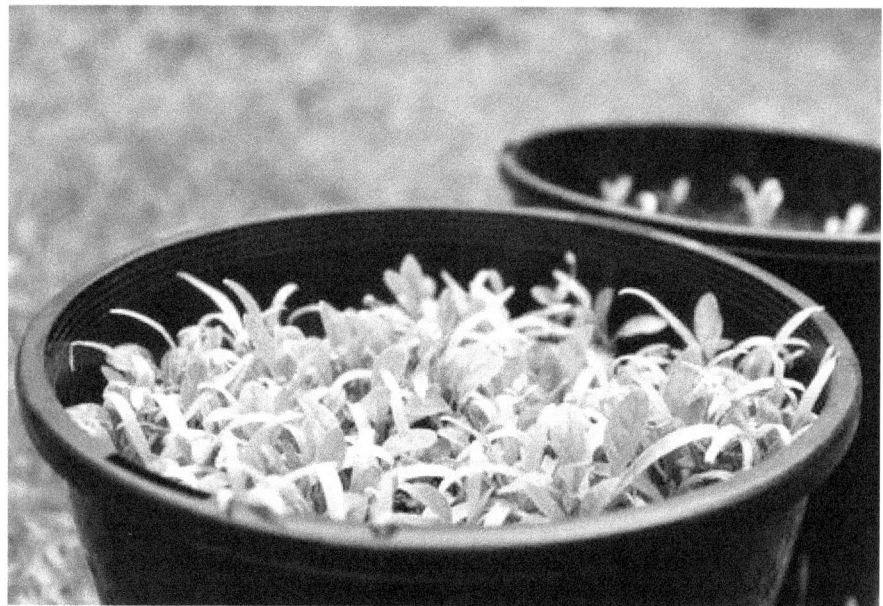

If you were brought up reading Popeye comics or watching Popeye cartoons, in the 30s and 40s, you may have noticed that the sailor man could not do without his spinach. This was to give him plenty of strength and energy. Also in popular literature, broccoli, spinach and other green vegetables have been given a bad name, because they are supposedly not worth eating.

Now that is a totally wrong misconception because spinach – Spinacia oleracea – is one of the most nutritious of greens available to mankind today. It is a native to southwestern Asia, from where it spread all over the world.

Spinach leaves are dark green in color, and a plant can grow up to 28 – 30 cm in height. Spinach normally likes a temperate climate, but you can also grow this plant in a place where the winter is going to be mild. Spinach does not like a snowy weather climate.

The fruit of the spinach is normally found in a lumpy and dry cluster, with a number of seeds in it. However, many gardeners do not allow the spinach to get to its fruition stage, because they would rather harvest the plant and sell it fresh, or eat it as a salad or cooked.

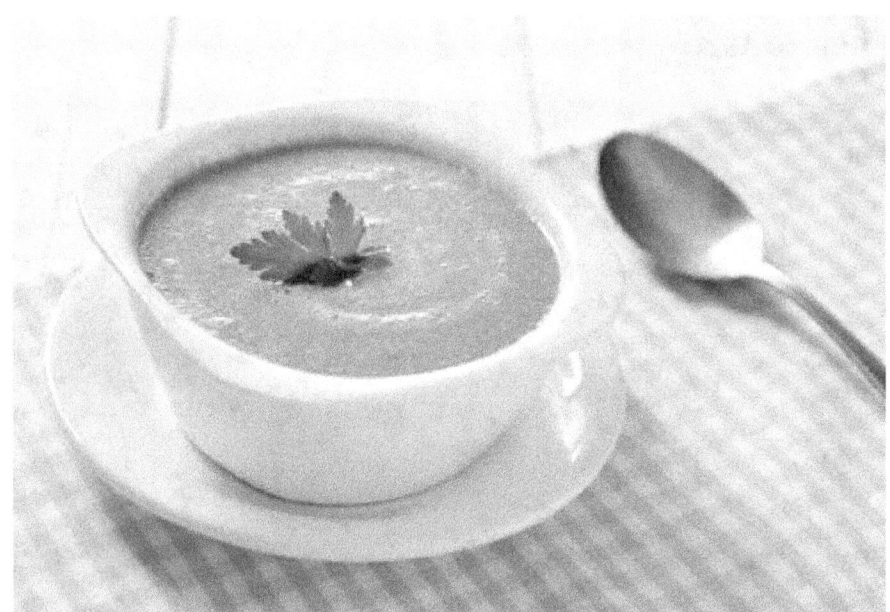

Spinach Soup – Healthy, Delicious and Nutritious!

In China, spinach is called the Persian vegetable, because it came to China from Persia hundreds of years ago through traders traveling on the Silk Route. But spinach was known to the Chinese as far back as 647 AD. 200 years later, Sicily was introduced to spinach by the Saracens. In Arabia, it was considered to be the chief of all the Leafy Greens- rais al buqul.

The Persians not only used spinach as a delicious, healthy dish, but they considered it to be extremely good for curing a number of ailments. Why not, because after all it was a good green leafy vegetable, easy to grow, even though it was a bit hard to digest when taken in large quantities. That is why if you want to eat lots of spinach, especially in the winter, always intersperse it with mouthfuls of orange slices. This is going to facilitate the absorption of iron into your system.

When to Grow Spinach

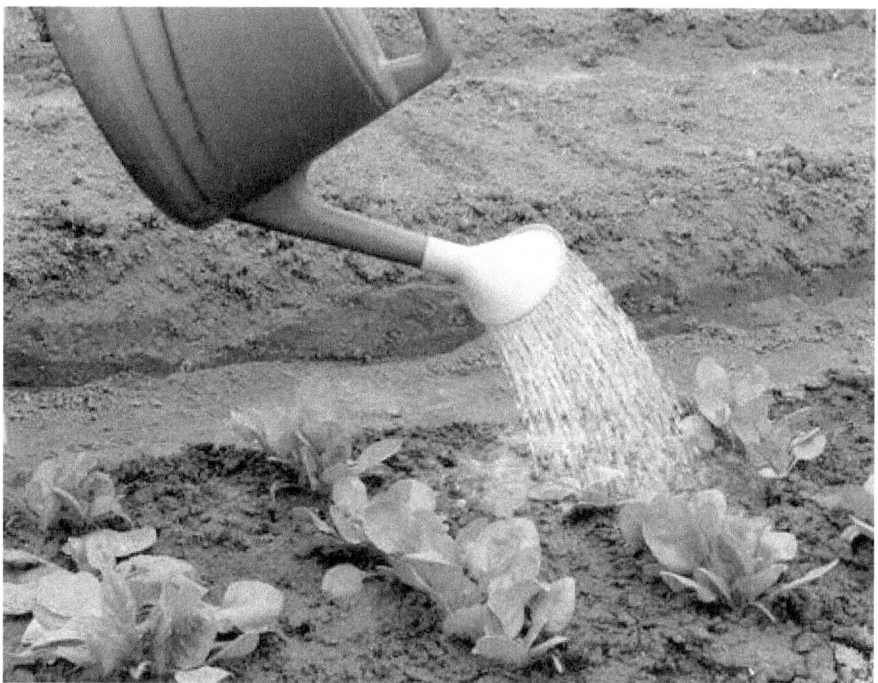

Spinach normally loves a temperate climate, so you can grow it anywhere, where you have plenty of sun. The USDA spinach growing hardiness zones range from three – nine.

Spinach can be grown in loamy, well fertilized and well watered land. The pH value of the soil has to be neutral.

Spinach seedlings are normally planted in the fall, winter and early spring, so that they can be harvested before the summer. Thanks to its versatile nutritious properties in nature, it can be eaten as a raw green salad, vegetable or in its cooked form.

It is a high provider source of vitamins, calcium and iron. When you compare it to other vegetables, you are going to see that it is one of the best available sources of important vitamins A, B, as well as vitamin C

Spinach usually does not like snowfall, but it does not mind the cold weather. That is why hot, nutritious spinach soup, and spinach food preparations are such a delight and blessing to all those people coming home after a cold day outside.

How to Plant Spinach

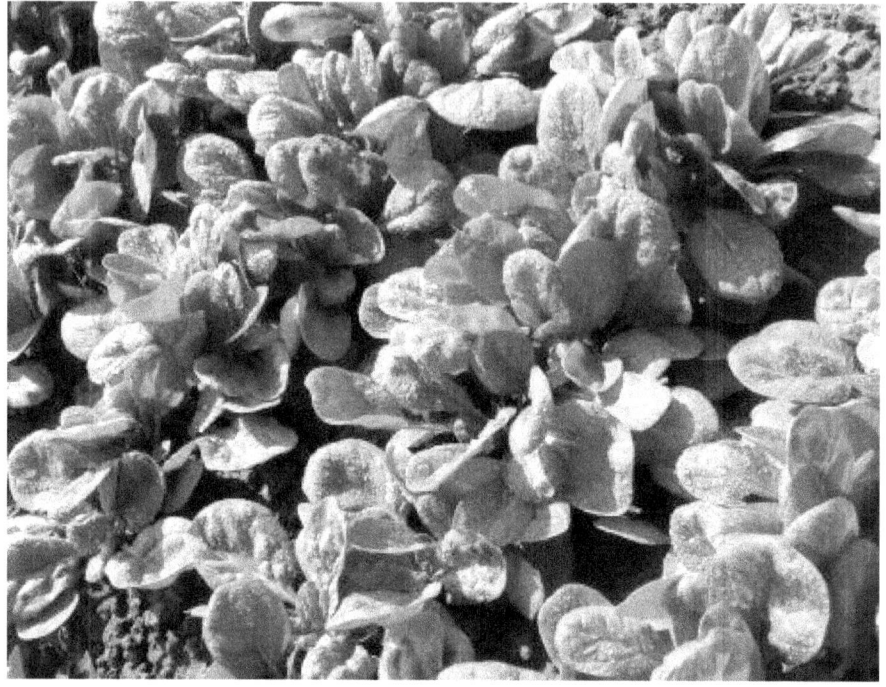

Spinach is such a versatile plant, that it can be grown anywhere in your backyard, either in beds, or in containers.

Before you plant spinach, you would want to prepare the bed, one week before hand. Use organic manure so that the soil has plenty of time to renew its nutrition content.

In many countries, a number of gardeners prepare the spinach beds in the fall, well fertilized with organic manure, so that the seeds can be sown in the winter or during early spring, after a winter thaw has melted.

If you are planting it in the summer or in the fall, you may want to look at the Malabar spinach variety or the New Zealand variety. That is, if you are living in a place where the winter is mild.

It is better to sow the seeds directly into the prepared area, because transplanting from seedlings is a traumatic experience for the baby spinach. So, sow, and allow them to grow. It is going to take six weeks for the spinach to reach harvesting stage so plant them keeping the weather in mind.

The soil should be well drained and the seeds should be planted in a site where you can get shaded areas, as well as full sun.

The seeds should be sown at a depth of half an inch to 1 inch. Cover them lightly with a thin layer of soil. You can either sprinkle all the seeds over a wide bed are a row or sow 12 of them to every foot. This is just about the space needed by a seedling to grow and flourish.

The temperature of the soil should to be 70°F. This facilitates the germination process.

Common spinach is more of a fall, winter and early spring plant. It does not grow in hot weather, especially Midsummer. You can continue successive plantings all through early spring, every couple of weeks so that you have a continuous supply of spinach.

If you want a crop in the fall, you need to plant your seeds in mid-August. An early spring sowing can be harvested in the fall, just before the coming of the winter. The best temperature for spinach to flourish is around 40°F. So if you find your spinach plants drooping in the winter, cover them with a layer of thick mulch. You may also want to protect them with cold protection frames. The new plants are going to need plenty of water, so make sure that you water them regularly.

Organic fertilizer, as I said is the best fertilizer for your plants, but you have to make sure you do not over fertilize the soil. If you think that there is a slow growth of your plants, do another fertilizing session with organic manure, when the plant has reached one third of its growth.

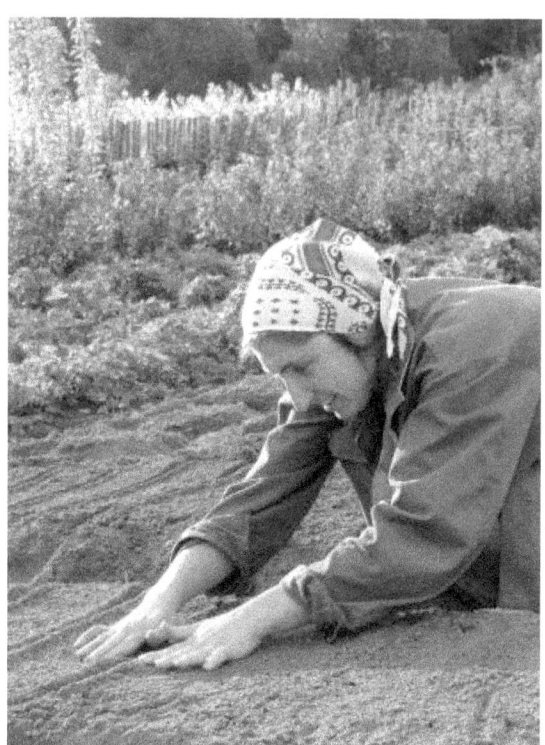

If you have sown the seeds by sprinkling, wait till they are 2 inches. Then, do thinning of the seedlings, at a distance of 3 to 4 inches between each plant. Do not bother more about your spinach, after this, except for watering because any other rough handling is going to damage the delicate roots.

If you have mulched the soil, remember to keep it moist. Spinach can survive the winter season to temperatures down to around 14°F. But protect your plants with a layer of mulch.

Harvesting Spinach

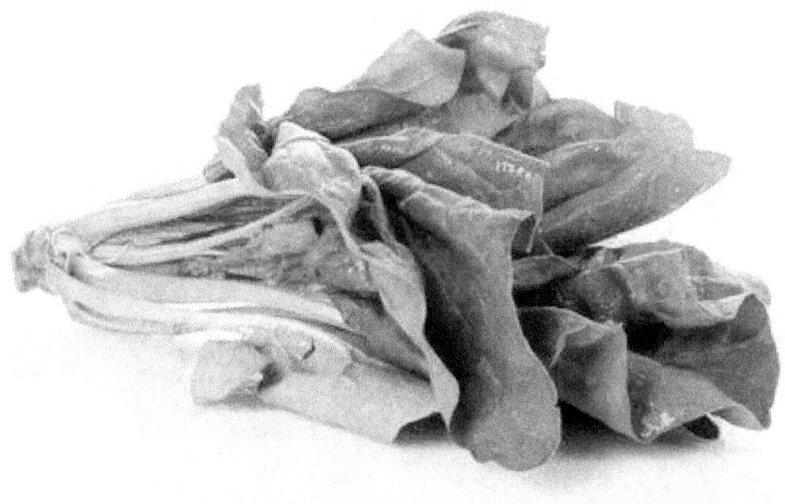

Make sure that the harvesting is done when the leaves have grown to a desired normal size. Do not wait for them to grow any larger. This is going to cause bitterness in the leaves, as the harvested plants reach maturity. It is much better to harvest them, with smaller leaves, than to harvest them with oversized and large a bitter leaves.

You can harvest them by cutting the plant off at the plant base, and leaving the root portion to be mulched back into the soil – or just picking off the leaves, layer by layer. This is going to give the inner layers of the plant more time to grow and develop. You can also harvest the whole spinach plant by uprooting it from its roots and clear the bed for another sowing.

Best Spinach Varieties

Winter Bloomsdale is a variety which is resistant to plant viruses, especially mosaic viruses and downy mildew. This along with Tyee is a good early spring, fall plant.

Spinach for Good Health

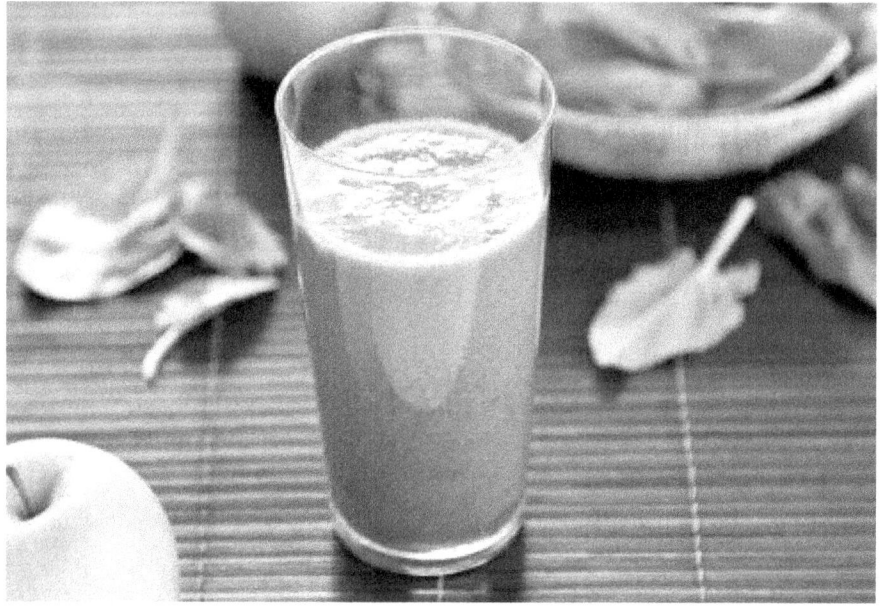

When we were children, we were encouraged to eat lots of spinach, because our elders said that it would give us rosy cheeks.[1] Nevertheless, we loved spinach, because first of all it was cooked in the traditional way which made it an excellent tasty, spicy dish for hungry little children, instead of being a soggy watery mess.

The second thing was that spinach could also be eaten raw, especially when crunched between bread-and-butter sandwiches, slices of egg, ham, cheese and pieces of lettuce – sometimes with a little bit of mayonnaise and sprinkle

---

[1] That was debatable because we were uniformly suntanned and sunburned throughout the year.

generously with salt, pepper, and spicy herbs. Not only was this combination delicious, but it was healthy and nutritious.

My grandmother always put a little pinch of baking powder or baking soda in the water while cooking spinach. This kept its color green.

Consider green leafy vegetables to be natural healers because of their chlorophyll content. In ancient times, anybody lethargic, pale looking and anaemic was immediately fed spinach, lettuce, seeds, dry and fresh fruit, sprouts, because this was the general health tonic.

Ancient power packed Spinach Health Tonic

Many people have forgotten about ancient natural healing remedies when people suffering from ailments were taken into hermitages and put on natural food diets.

This recipe calls for these green leafy vegetables to be chopped up in equal quantities, and drunk down – 2 cups every day.

I am telling you all about the leafy vegetables easily available in your nearest organic vegetable store. These include broccoli, spinach, kale, chard, lettuce , amaranth, asparagus, bok choy, mint, parsley, cabbage and celery. In the East, we use mustard leaves – which has a sharp taste – water spinach, and kohlrabi. Consider this power pack to be your safeguard against infections, healing your body and rejuvenating you.

Try drinking this mixture every day for three weeks. If you do not see a distinct, establishing and amazing improvement in your health, including rosy cheeks, well, you will need to see a doctor because there is something distinctively seriously wrong with your system.

For all of us who have acquired a subconscious autosuggestion of all green leafy vegetables are yuck during childhood, the mere thought of drinking green juice in such large quantities is going to make you shudder. Let me give you one suggestion to make this more palatable. For your first cup in the morning add some chunks of pineapple. For your second cup in the evening, add another of your favorite fruits and even a little bit of honey.

You will be pleasantly surprised at how different these food textures and taste combinations can taste.

I got into this habit of drinking green vegetable juices as a child, because luckily I had parents who were very sensible about eating and drinking. They encouraged us to eat greens and fruit, without ever telling us, "eat this, because it is a good thing for you." If they had said that, we would immediately have turned our noses up at that particular food, and never eaten it again.

Instead, my father used inverse psychology. He would make up something "experimental" for himself, with a little bit of this green and a little bit of that green and a little bit of this fruit, and a little bit of that herb and then say, "all right, I am trying it out, because I am a grown-up. I do not know whether kids would enjoy this as much as we grown-ups would enjoy it."

That would immediately make us very enthusiastic and eager about trying that particular juice mixture. In fact, we clamored for it. He would then be very reluctant and tell us, "okay then, you can just try half a cup. Who knows, you may not like it," all the time, eyeing the mixture with a look that clearly said, "all the better for me, if you do not like it. I get to finish it off."

What half a cup, we wanted a full cup. Sometimes we wanted a glass, because hey it was tasty. And that is why, we as adults now are reaping the benefits of those healthy foods eaten during childhood, with lots of thanks to a sensible parent.

One of these mixtures was spinach juice, mint, and pieces of fruit. We loved the minty taste. We felt ourselves real Brave Hearts because we were drinking full glasses of spinach juice and well, lots of fruit would do for us every day, anytime.

So you can see that if a parent does not create some sort of green phobia in the mind of the child, just because he himself has not learned good eating habits from his parents, children are more open to sensible suggestions of drinking healthy foods in juice form.

Problems Caused Due to Radiation Exposure

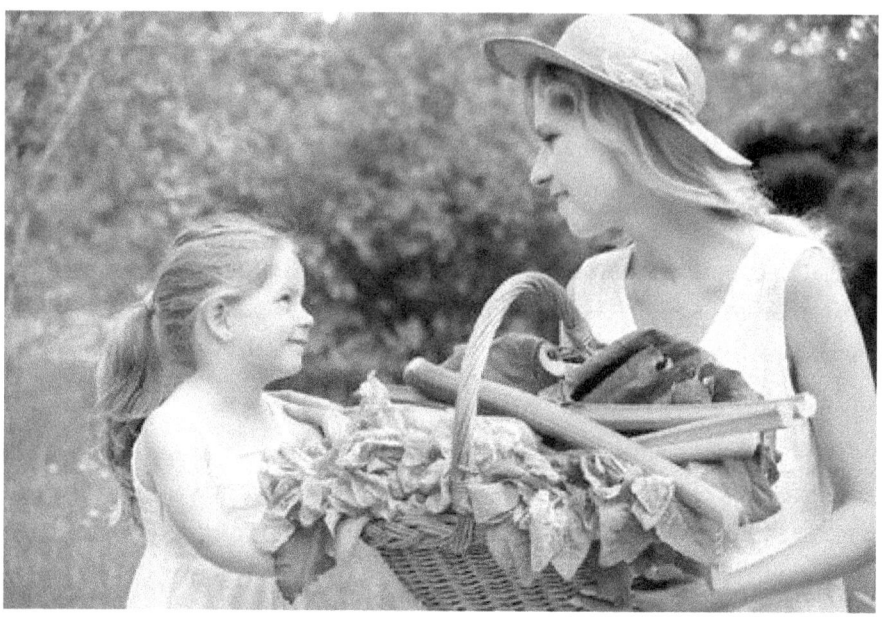

Green leafy vegetables – healthy for you. They also prevent Radiation problems

Do you know that all over the world people are worrying about radiation exposure, which is one of the reasons why so many people are suffering from skin ailments? Many people are scared that sitting in front of a computer is going to expose them to radiation. [That incidentally, is a mischievous and baseless rumor started by somebody who intends to market an expensive beauty product which protects you from computer radiation in the future. Well, my wicked brain has thought up this idea; the moment somebody markets it, I am going to say I told you so.]

Anyway, eating dark green leafy vegetables have been guaranteed to give you protection against radiation. This research was done in 1962 by Dr. Doris Calloway. At that time, the radiation scare was minimal. The 2020s has that scare escalating a hundredfold. So protect yourself from carcinogen creating components in the atmosphere by increasing the amount of green leafy vegetables, full of good chlorophyll in your diet right now.

Apart from this, spinach has many other benefits, which have been known to people down the centuries.

Benefits of a regular Spinach Diet

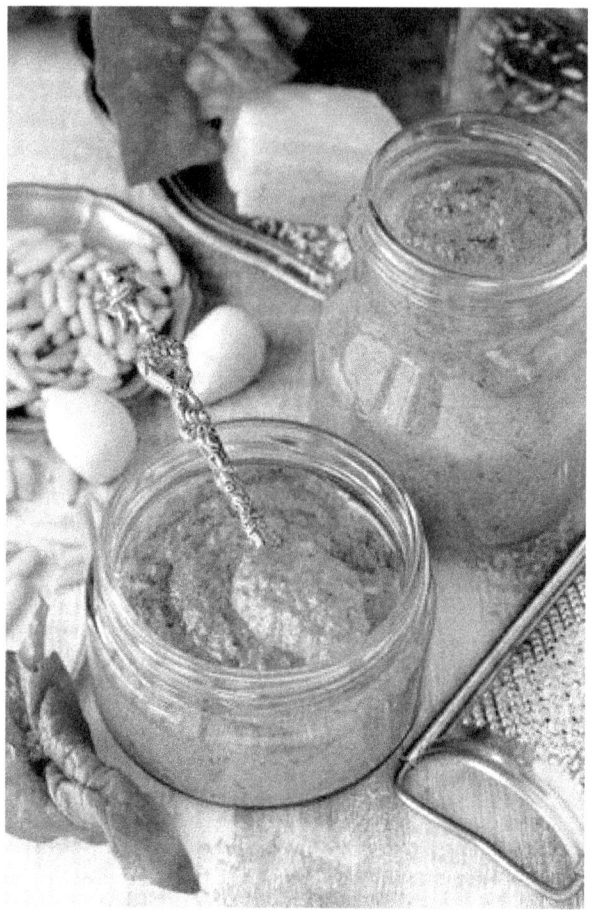

A spinach pesto is an excellent addition to your diet.[2]

Spinach has an important ingredient called Folacin. It is a vitamin. According to a number of doctors and researchers, folacin has been one of the major natural vitamins, which prevent birth defects like brain damage or cleft palate or even

---

[2] http://www.thekitchn.com/how-to-make-perfect-pesto-every-time-cooking-lessons-from-the-kitchn-175471

Instead of the greens given here in this URL, try spinach.

poor learning abilities in a child. That is why an expectant mother is always recommended healthy doses of spinach in the East. This also improves the performance of the liver.

A number of cancers can be prevented by eating spinach. These cancers include pancreatic cancer, cervical cancer and lung cancer.

Body cell reproduction, rejuvenation and growth is greatly enhanced with spinach. It is also considered to be good for the continuous creation of hemoglobin in your blood.[3]

So which is going to give us the most benefit? Cooked spinach or spinach eaten raw?

---

[3] Thus the rosy cheeks! But I can safely reiterate that spinach juice is excellent for your skin, keeping it glowing, and healthy. You may also find your eyes shining more, after drinking a lot of spinach juice.

Spinach in Your Cuisine

Remember that all vitamin B products, especially folic acid – folacin – are quite delicate. They are destroyed on exposure to heat, like other vitamins. Also, many of us have a tendency of cooking green leafy vegetables until they are a solid mass. And then we grind them and fry them and serve them up.

This cooking procedure lessens the natural powerful potency of the spinach. Also, many of us boil these vegetables before and send the water in which it has been cooked down the drain, instead of drinking it up[4] or using that water to make up the gravy portion of the cooked dish.

So I would suggest getting your spinach, fresh, and eating it as soon as possible. Putting it in the fridge is good only if you intend to eat it while it is still fresh. Otherwise you are going to have yellowish, soggy, wilted leaves.

Spinach leaves have oxalic acid in them. Oxalic acid has been given lots of bad publicity throughout the years, but it is as I said, bad publicity. Oxalic acid is one of the necessary ingredients which you need to keep your system working properly. Raw spinach is excellent to cure problems like tumors. This is a fact well known to traditional healers. Asparagus also has oxalic acid. So as far as possible, eat asparagus and spinach, raw, to get the most out of them, especially the high potassium content.

---

[4] Like I do. Delicious, but an acquired taste, especially in spinach and mustard and other greens. For mustard water, I have to take a deep breath first before gulping it down.

Choosing the Best Spinach

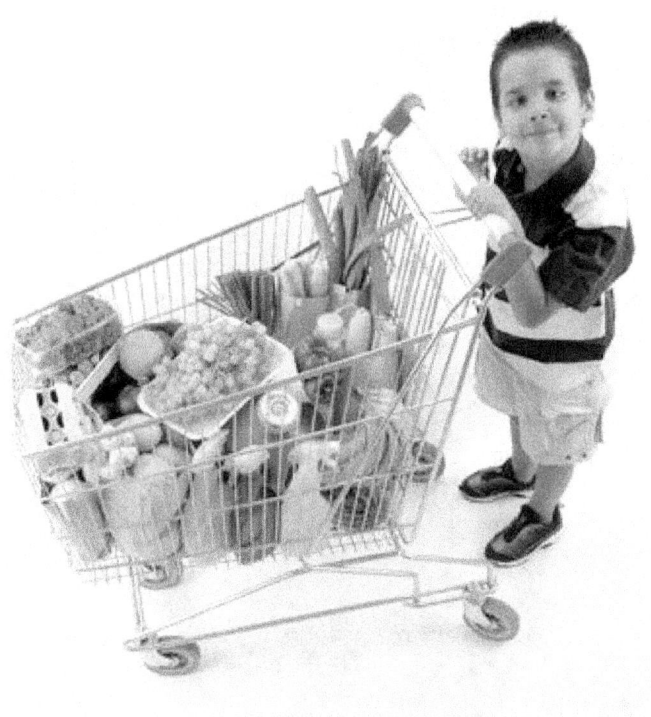

So where is the spinach?

If you are plucking spinach from your garden patch, well, the leaves are going to be fresh, green and healthy. But when you are shopping for spinach, look for spinach, which does not have any sort of yellow twinges. That means it has over matured, and the leaves have over jumped their healthy and healing qualities.

Do not buy plants which are wilting. Organic plants are best. Unfortunately, it is the tendency for a number of farmers to spray all their vegetables with terrible poisonous toxins. So you will need to detoxify the spinach.

There is a company in America, called NutriBiotic. It makes a non-toxic soap in a liquid form. I was astonished at the thought that one would want to wash vegetables with a soap, to get rid of the toxins, but unfortunately that is what needs to be done nowadays. The liquid grapefruit extract made by the same company is also excellent to detoxify and disinfect vegetables and fruit. This is done by mixing anywhere between 15 – 20 drops of this extract in a gallon of water.

Dump all your vegetables in that water disinfecting soak. Allowed to stand for 20 minutes. Then allow to drain. Make sure the leaves retain a little bit of moisture before you pack them away. Spinach leaves should not touch each other when you are storing them away in your refrigerator. Otherwise, you are going to get a yellow wilted mass. They are going to last up to two days in your fridge.

If you are getting spinach, fresh from a farm make sure that it has been washed thoroughly with saltwater before you decide to eat it. If you wash it and preserve it, the natural decaying process is going to be speeded up. If you are picking off the leaves in your garden, just do not wash them vigorously, because you know that you have not used any chemical toxins or poisonous pesticides.

Quick Steamed Spinach

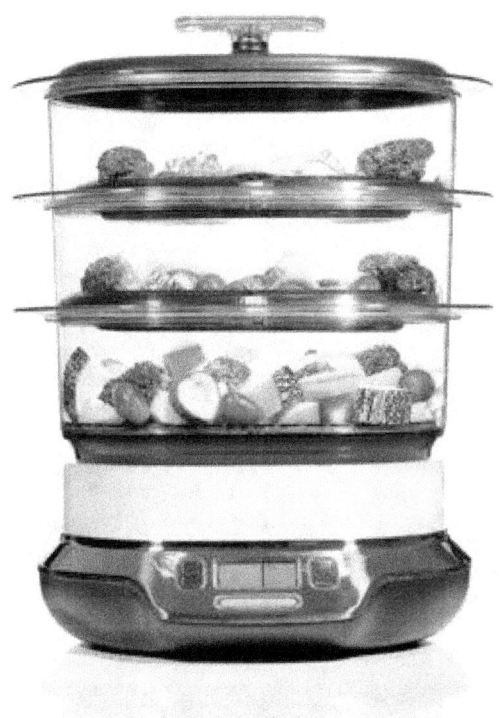

A steam cooker is excellent for steaming any number of vegetables at the same time.

This is what I normally do, so that all the natural goodness of the spinach is retained. This is when I want to cook spinach instead of using it as a salad. I use a vegetable steamer which has a basket in it. The leaves are put on the basket and placed above the water in the steamer. Two minutes steaming is going to give me excellent steamed spinach. I then grind it and place it in my freezer, to eat whenever wanted.

For use, I break off chunks of frosted spinach, and allow to defrost. The rest of the spinach goes back into the freezer.

Introduction to Saag

If you are in South Asia, and have entered a hotel, where the menu keeps talking about Saag – with a number of vegetables, including peas, cauliflowers, potatoes, cottage cheese, and meat added to the saag; you pronounce the way it is written with an a: sound-you know that you are going to be fed a leaf-based spicy mixture, made up of spinach.

 This is eaten with the local bread – roti – or rice. Traditional Saag is normally made up of spinach and mustard leaf in equal measures, along with some amaranth leaves, if available. Any sort of green added to the mixture is equally welcome.

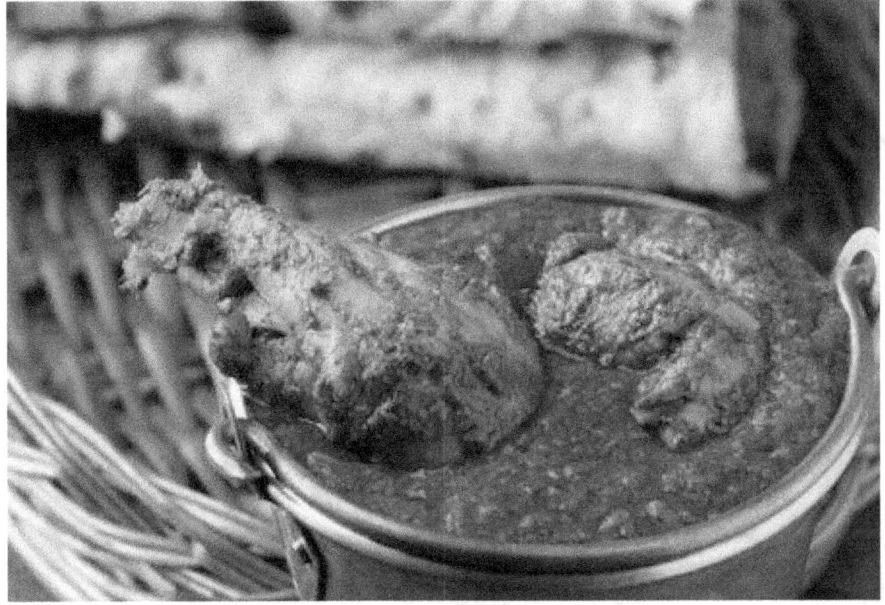

Saag can be eaten as a main dish, by itself, but here it is the base for chicken. It can also be the base for fish, cottage cheese and potatoes. Consider this word to be the catchall cuisine term for any mixture of green leafy vegetables ground into a spicy mixture, and flavored with a lot of herbs, cooked and garnished with onions, fresh, homemade butter, green chilies and served piping hot.

You can also make fenugreek leaves into a Saag. In many parts of the northern portions of the Indian subcontinent, any meat, which is to be added to a saag base is marinated overnight, and then cooked in a tandoor like chicken or lamb. It is then added to the cooked Saag, thus combining two delicious and spicy textures together.

Traditional Saag is normally made up with a mixture of spinach leaves and mustard leaves. This is normal winter fare, eaten every afternoon in the majority of the villages in the northern part of the Indian subcontinent. It is then washed down with buttermilk and then the happy diner goes off to sleep like an Anaconda for about three hours. This is to facilitate the digestion of that nutritious and delicious meal. You cannot eat this, if you have work to do in the afternoon, chained to your desk. Unless of course, you have somebody to nudge you awake, when you keep dropping off to sleep.

Traditional Saag

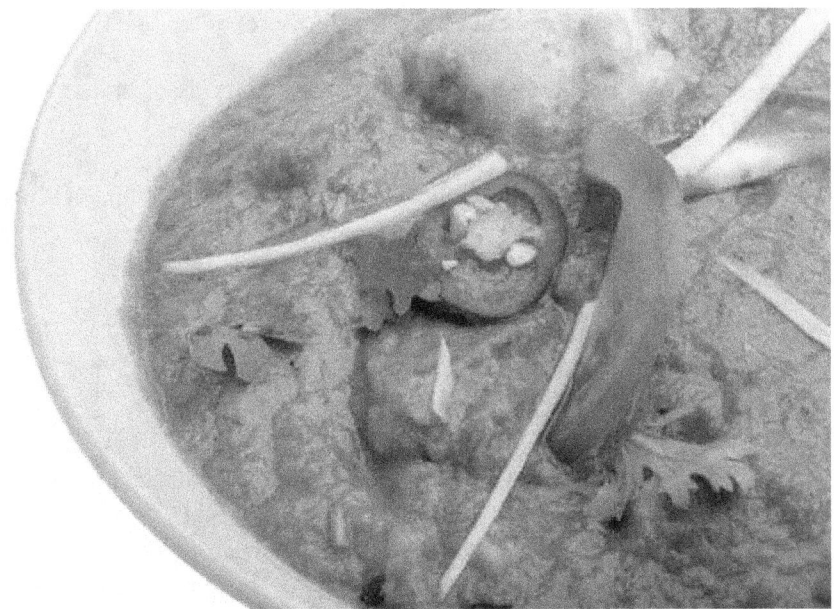

Potatoes have been added to the traditional saag base.

This is made up with 2 pounds of spinach leaves, 1 ounce of clarified butter, half a teaspoonful of salt, one teaspoonful of ground ginger powder and a pinch of sugar.

Clarified butter is known as desi ghee. It is made by taking 1 pound of best butter and melting in a heavy pan with an asbestos mat underneath. Heat this to just below simmering point, and maintain this heat for about 40 minutes. Increase the time for a larger quantity of butter.

Much of the moisture in the butter will have evaporated and the impurities are going to sink to the bottom of the pan. Pour off the concentrated clarified butter carefully, straining through several thicknesses of Muslin cloth.

If kept in a cool place, this clarified butter is going to last for a year or so without turning rancid.

It is considered to be the best of all cooking fats – and of course the most expensive – in many parts of Asia. That is because it can be heated to a higher temperature than even the best olive oil or mustard oil. For this reason, it is the best, most popular chosen frying medium. It is going to give you the most crisp fried results. The high temperature prevents the secret of the fact inside the food.

You may want to sear meat in clarified butter prior to frying or braising, in a meat-based dish.

So now that we have our clarified butter, let us go back to making healthy spinach saag.

This is done by washing the spinach and shredding it very fine. Put it in a pan with the melted butter and less than 2 tablespoons full of water, salt, sugar and ginger.

Mix well to stop. Cover and leave on very high heat for two minutes, then on medium heat until it is soft and all the moisture has evaporated. This is going to take 25 to 30 minutes. Stir once or twice during this period.

Uncover, mix well and leave uncovered on low heat for three or four minutes before serving.

Now that we have made the basic spinach base, it can be made into

Dry Spinach and Potatoes

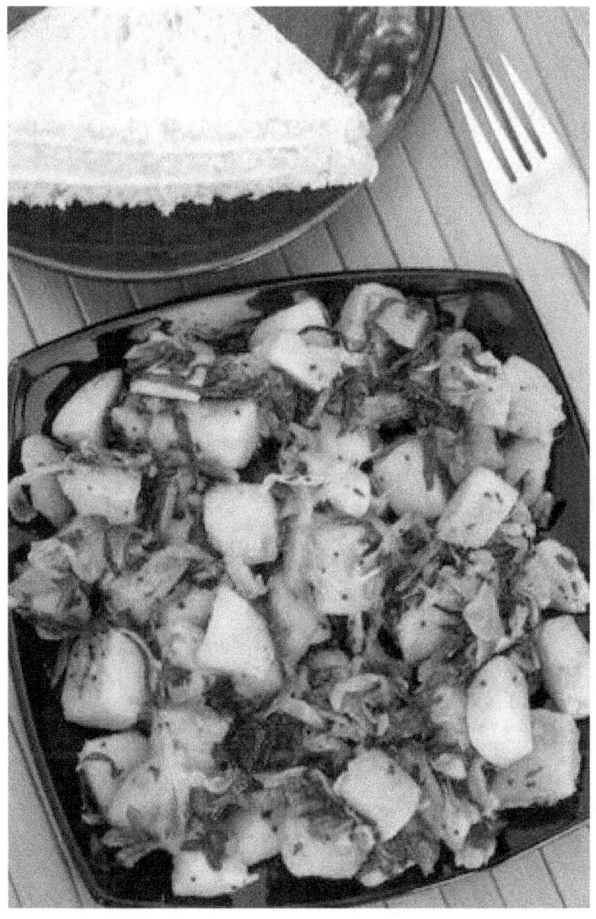

You can either use the spinach base, made above, and follow the recipes for cooking potatoes and adding it to this mixture, or you can try it from the very beginning.

For this you need two and a half pounds of spinach, 2 ounces of clarified butter, 1 pound of potatoes, two large onions, sliced thin, one crushed clove of garlic, one teaspoonful of coriander, ¼ teaspoonful of apricot, one minced green pimento, one crushed cardamom, 1 inch piece of green ginger, cut into julienne strips, and ¾ teaspoonful of salt.

Wash the spinach well. Boil, then simmer in a little salted water until it is tender, about 12 minutes. Peel and cut the potatoes into harms or quarters. Drain the spinach well and chop it very fine. Keep aside. Prepare the aromatics on medium heat.

In a heavy saucepan, heat the butter. Add the ginger and fry until it is crisp.

Add the potatoes, garlic, onions, paprika, coriander, crushed cardamom and pimento. Leave without stirring for just one minute. Now stir lightly and allow to cook for another minute. Then stir and fry until the potatoes are well browned.

Now, raise the heat to very high, and the cooked spinach, I pinch more of salt, and Marston, with half a pint of water.

Stir over very high heat. Close the lid and steam over low heat until the potatoes are tender.

Stir and dry of any remaining moisture, leaving the spinach and potatoes well-buttered.

You can eat this dish without potatoes if you want. Garnish with pieces of lemon, raw onions and green chilies.

Lamb with Spinach

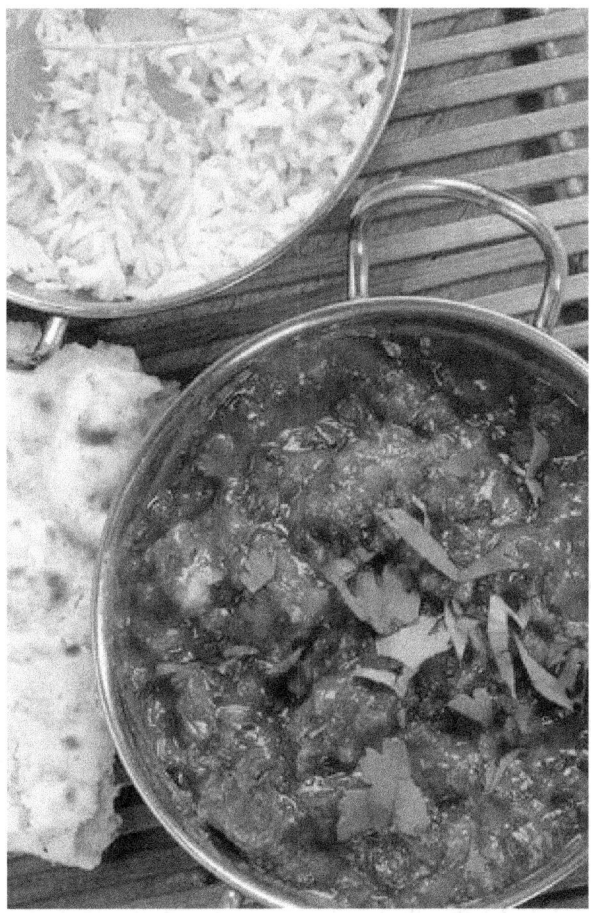

This is a traditional dish very popular in Western restaurants. But you may find the dish heavily spiced or made up with cooking oils, instead of clarified butter. That is because the traditional dish is very rich, and it is normally eaten on special occasions. Of course you can have it every day for dinner, if you have a very active lifestyle and can manage to digest all that spinach, meat and butter.

For this you need two pounds of spinach, 1 ½ pounds of deboned lamb, 2 ounces of clarified butter, six grated shallots, 2 inches of fresh ginger, three crushed cardamoms, 11/4 tablespoons ground coriander seeds, 2 teaspoons full of turmeric, one green chili, ¼ teaspoons full of paprika, one tablespoonful of mustard seeds, and ¼ teaspoons full of salt. Apart from

this, you will need to make a garlic infusion made with four cloves of garlic crushed and steeped for 30 minutes in 4 tablespoons full of warm water. Also, you will need 4 large tablespoons full of yogurt.

Dry fry all the aromatics on a griddle, and then chop or pound them accordingly. Wash the spinach well and steep in cold water for several hours. This is done in areas, where you do not have access to detoxifying soap, which is a modern product! And as we are making traditional saag, we are using the methods used by our grandmothers down the ages.

Drain, chop very fine, cover and put aside.

Now cube the Lamb and fry in half of the butter with the cardamoms and three quarters of the coriander until it has been browned all over.

Add grated shallots, and continue frying and stirring continuously until the shallots are dark gold in color.

Mix in the fresh ginger, which has been cut into julienne strips and fry together for about a minute.

Now begin adding the spices and the rest of the herbs, beginning with turmeric, the rest of the coriander and the green chili, which has been made into slivers. Traditionally, people like this dish hot, but if you do not want it hot, you can remove the seeds. The seeds have the chili hot factor in them.

Stir and fry together for another minute without scorching. Now add the paprika and stir and fry for a few seconds, scraping the bottom of the pan. Fry the mustard seeds, using just enough of butter to grease the pan and when the seeds begin to crackle and snap, add these to the meat.

Stir and aromatize with the garlic infusion. Raise the heat and stir vigorously for about one minute.

Some people normally add one tablespoonful of roasted, ground poppy seeds, to the mixture here at this stage of cooking, but I consider it to be optional. Nevertheless, if you enjoy seeds in a rich, delicious preparation, go right ahead.

Now, top with chopped spinach, season with salt, moisten with the whipped yogurt and cover well.

For one minute, raising the heat and shaking the Wok or casserole, five or six times, so that the food can be cooked evenly.[5]

Lower the heat, uncover and mix well. Cover again and cook over the lowest heat until the spinach is velvet-ty and the meat is very tender. Moisten with ¾ cups of water, then stir and cook over medium heat, and dry off all the moisture.

Now, cover, and give the casserole a last moment cook for 20 more minutes in a gentle oven. [6]

You can also place live charcoals on top and heat over an asbestos mat over heat or a flame. Garnish with strips of onions, pieces of chopped chilies, coriander and serve piping hot with either boiled rice or bread.

My father cannot resist adding a little bit of cream, to this mixture, even though it is very rich, just before serving. He places the cream in his serving plate and then pours the hot dish over it. One hearty stir, a little bit of chopped onions and chilies, and lunch is served. So they should show you that this dish is not for people who are obsessed with weight watching.

---

[5] If you are fortunate enough to see this dish being cooked in the open air, in a market, you are going to notice that the cook insouciantly picks up the Wok, with two pieces of cloth, raises it above the fire, and stirs it in clockwise and anticlockwise motions, a number of times. This is showmanship of the highest order. He then plops it back on the fire, and goes back to scolding his helper for being a lazy lump, especially when hungry people are clamoring for lunch or dinner.

[6] Diehards are going to be using a tandoor for this last cooking stage. You can consider a tandoor to be a Dutch oven.

Conclusion

This book has introduced you to the magic of spinach, one of the most nutritious of green leafy vegetables available to you as a bountiful gift of nature today. So make spinach a part and parcel of your daily diet, and see the immediate improvement in your health.

Along with spinach, more green leafy vegetables added to your daily diet are going to be very beneficial to you in the long run, especially when you start enjoying eating greens when you are young.

Live Long and Prosper!

Author Bio

Dueep Jyot Singh is a Management and IT Professional who managed to gather Postgraduate qualifications in Management and English and Degrees in Science, French and Education while pursuing different enjoyable career options like being an hospital administrator, banker, IT,SEO and HRD Database Manager/ trainer, movie , radio and TV scriptwriter, theatre artiste and public speaker, lecturer in French, Marketing and Advertising, ex-Editor of Hearts On Fire (now known as Solstice) Books Missouri USA, advice columnist and cartoonist, publisher and Aviation School trainer, ex- moderator on Medico.in, banker, student councilor ,travelogue writer … among other things!

One fine morning, she decided that she had enough of killing herself by Degrees and went back to her first love -- writing. It's more enjoyable! She already has 48 published academic and 14 fiction- in- different- genre books under her belt.

When she is not designing websites or making Graphic design illustrations for clients , she is browsing through old bookshops hunting for treasures, of which she has an enviable collection – including R.L. Stevenson, O.Henry, Dornford Yates, Maurice Walsh, De Maupassant, Victor Hugo, Sapper, C.N. Williamson, "Bartimeus" and the crown of her collection- Dickens "The Old Curiosity Shop," and so on… Just call her "Renaissance Woman") - collecting herbal remedies, acting like Universal Helping Hand/Agony Aunt, or escaping to her dear mountains for a bit of exploring, collecting herbs and plants and trekking.

Our books are available at
1. Amazon.com
2. Barnes and Noble
3. Itunes
4. Kobo
5. Smashwords
6. Google Play Books

Check out some of the other JD-Biz Publishing books
Gardening Series on Amazon

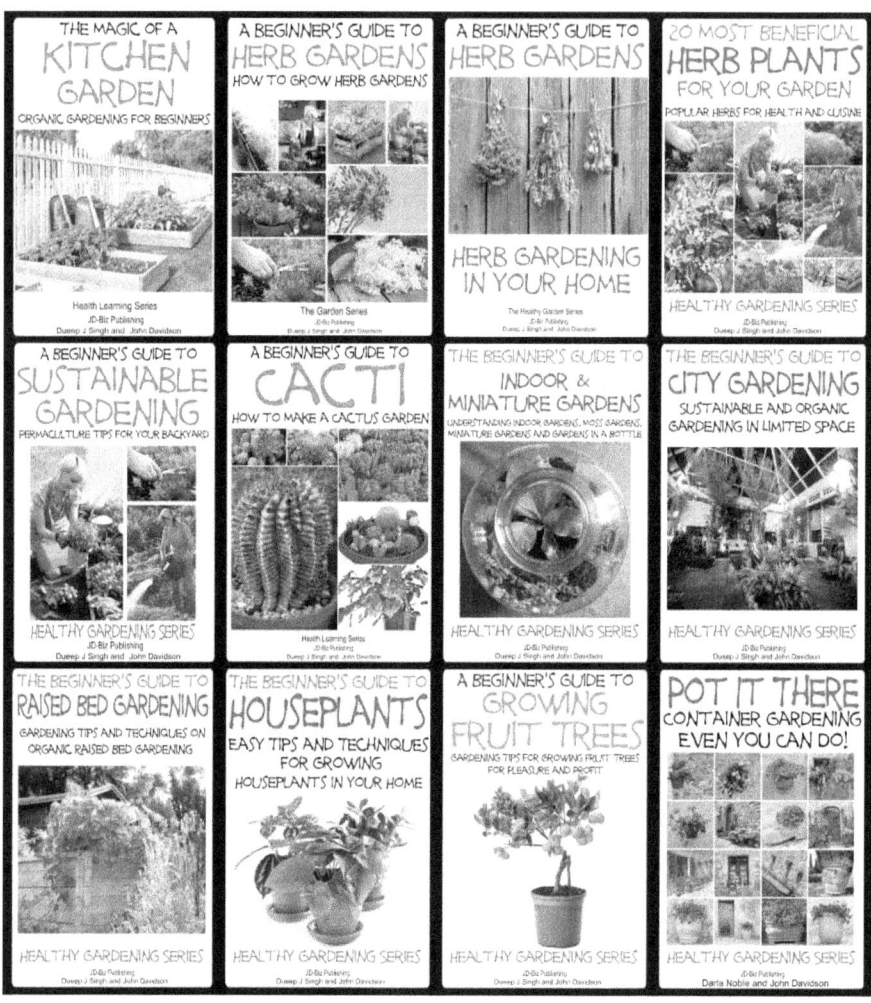

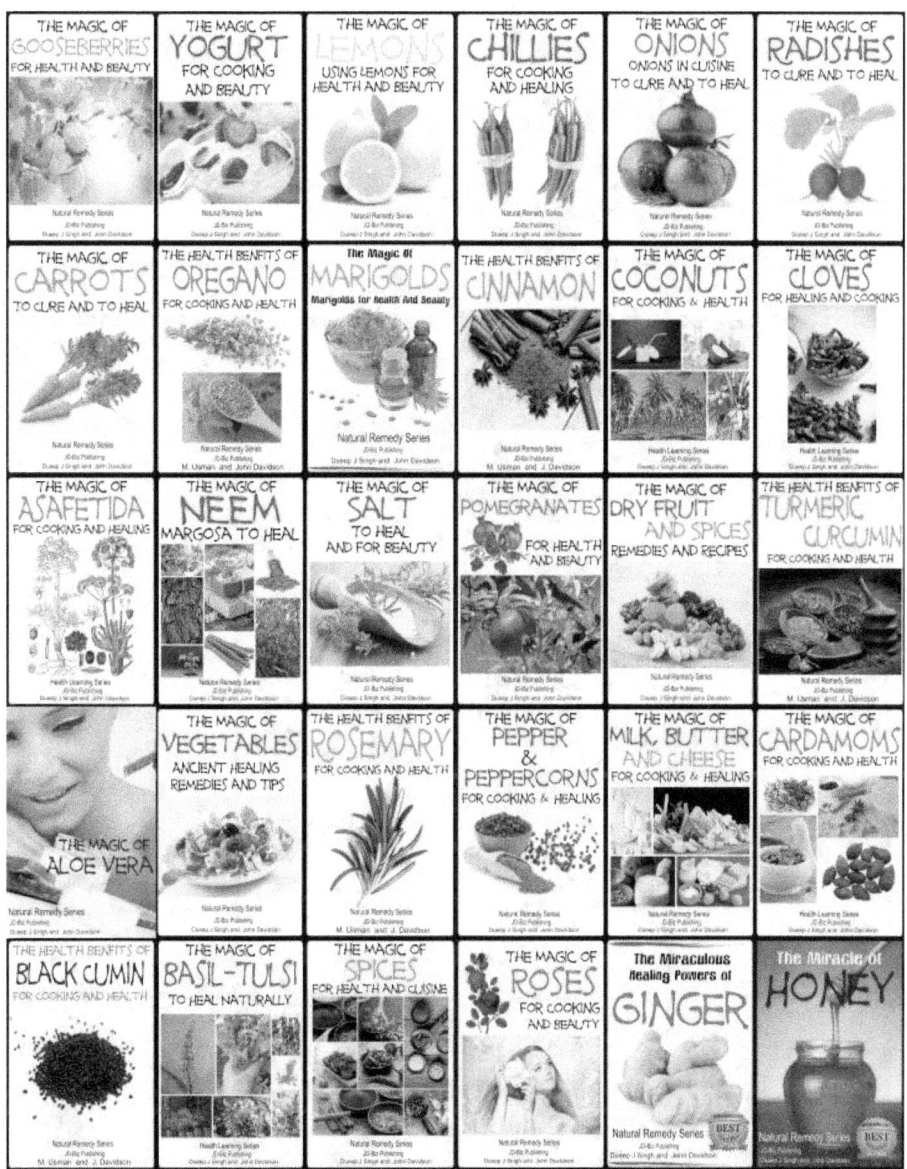

Country Life Books

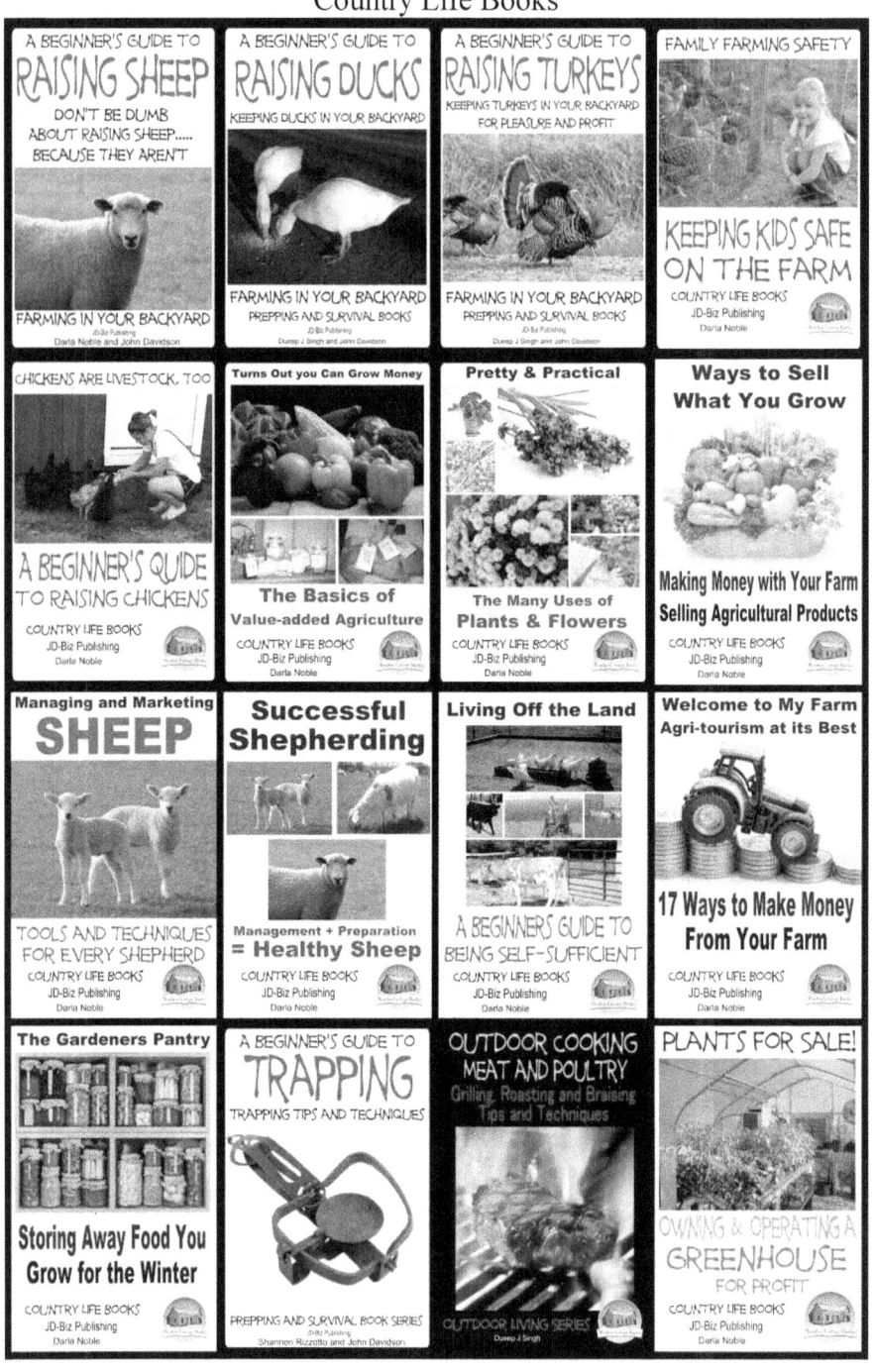

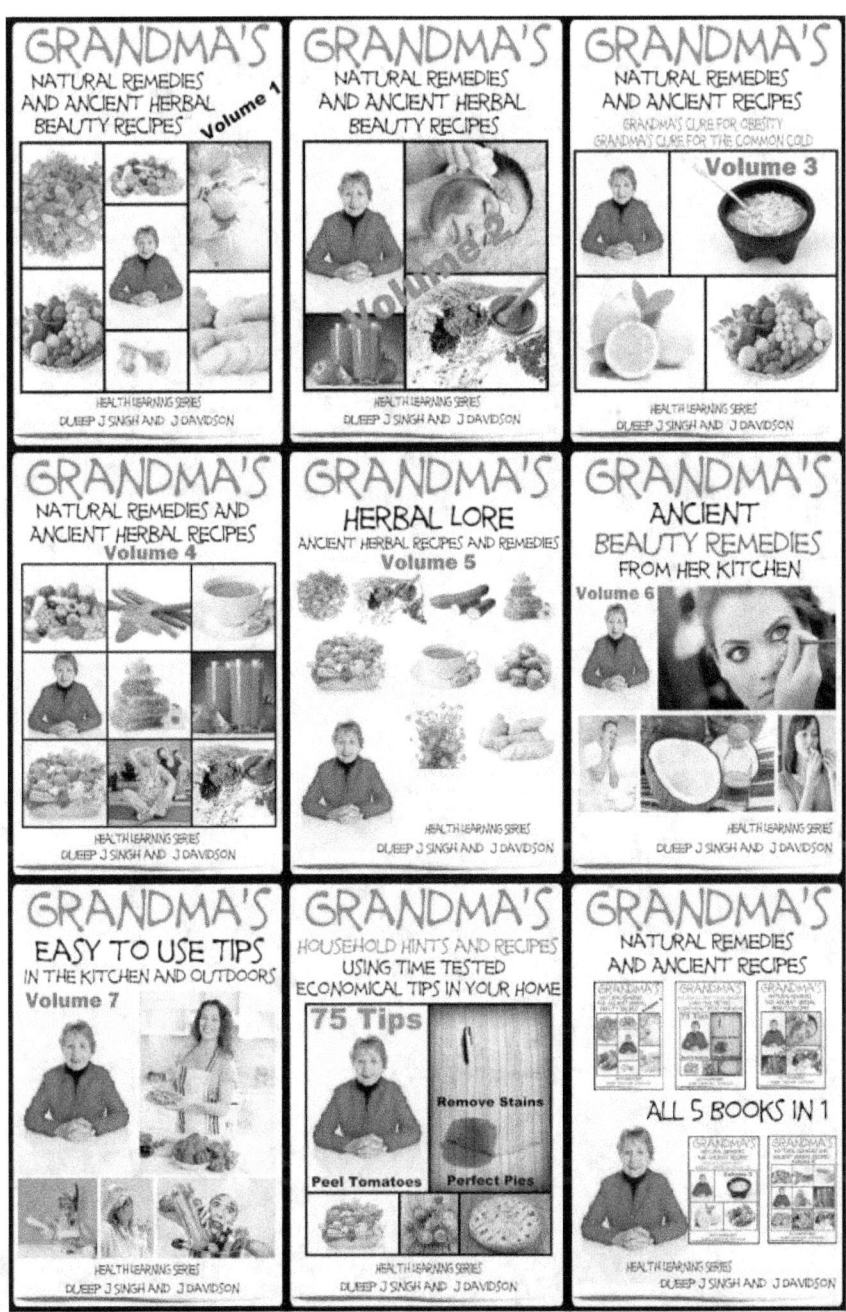

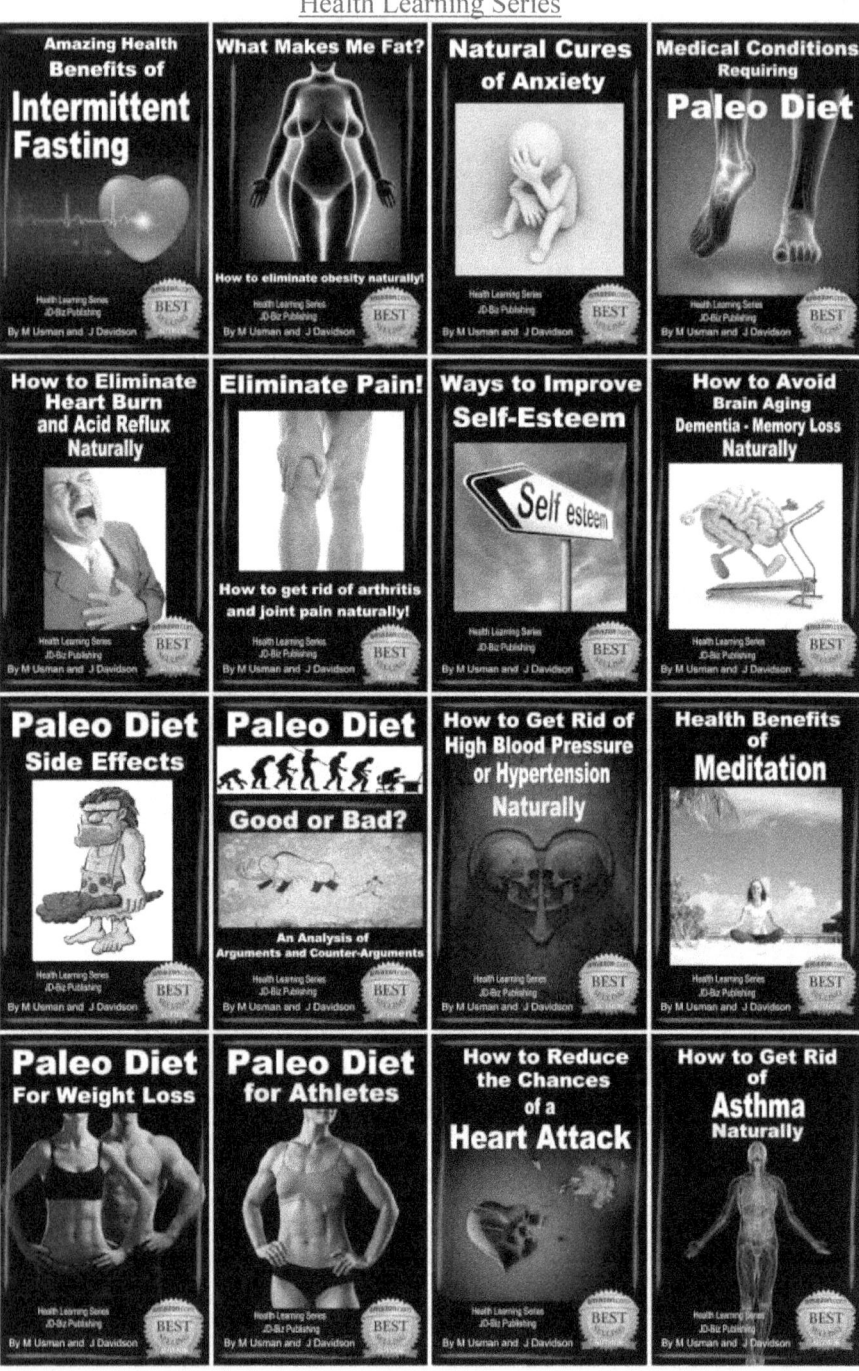

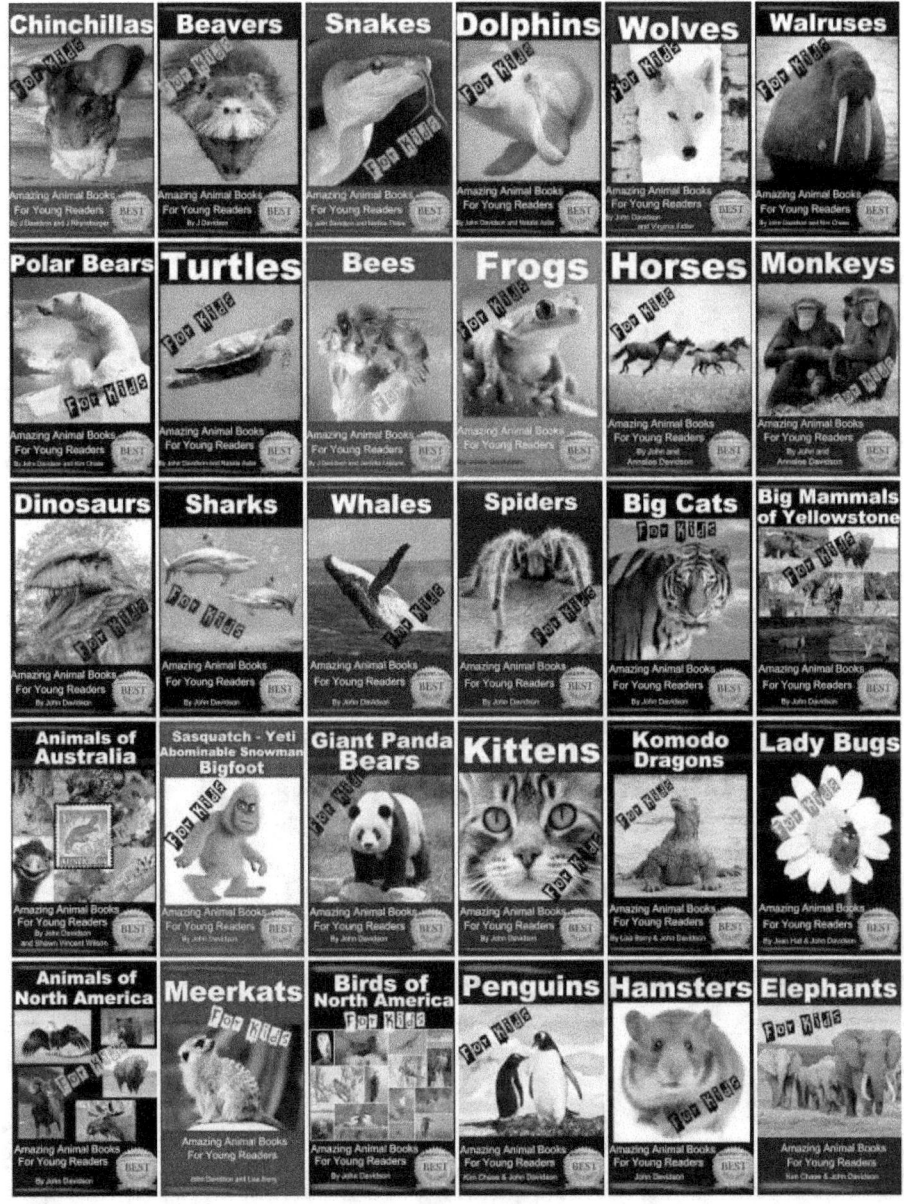

Learn To Draw Series

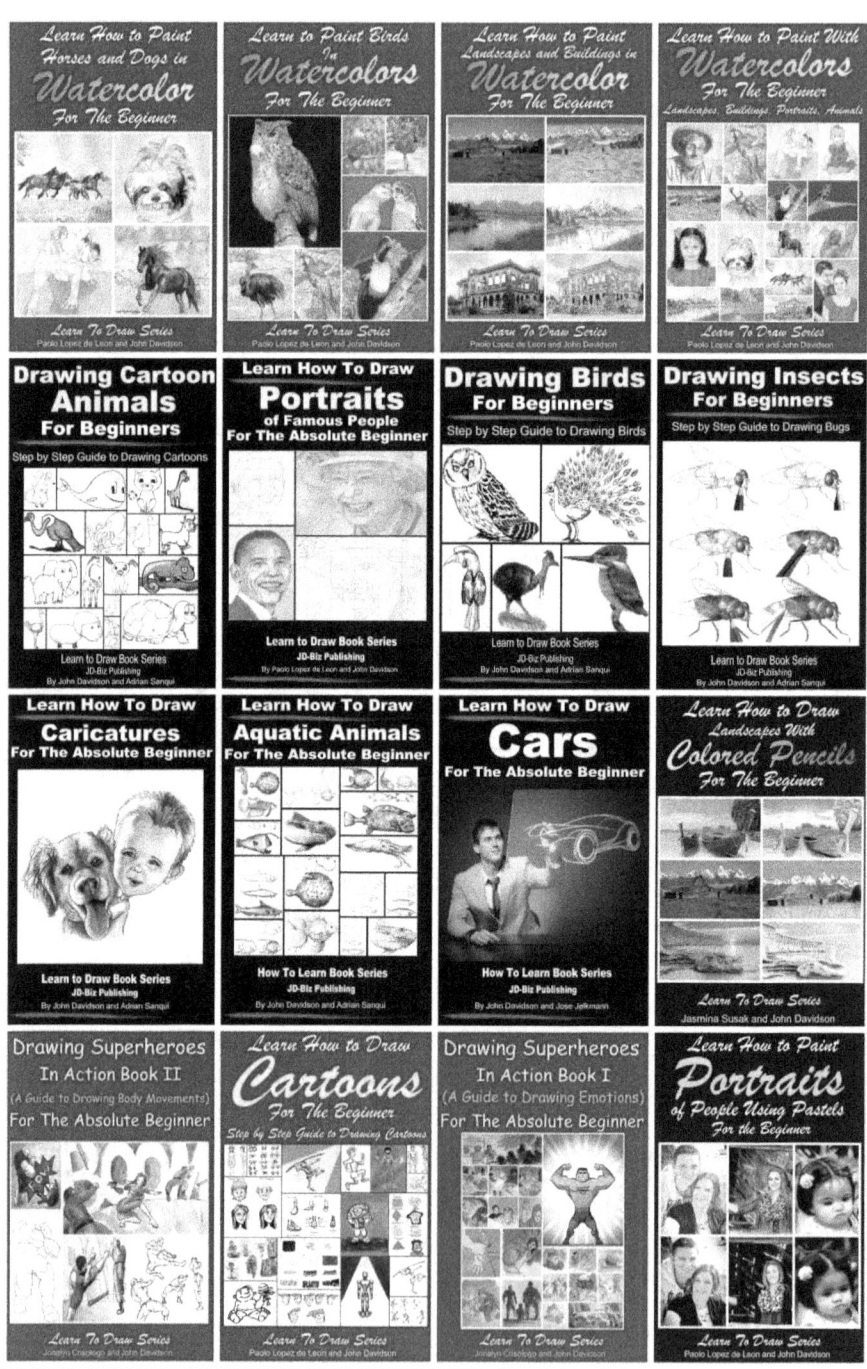

How to Build and Plan Books

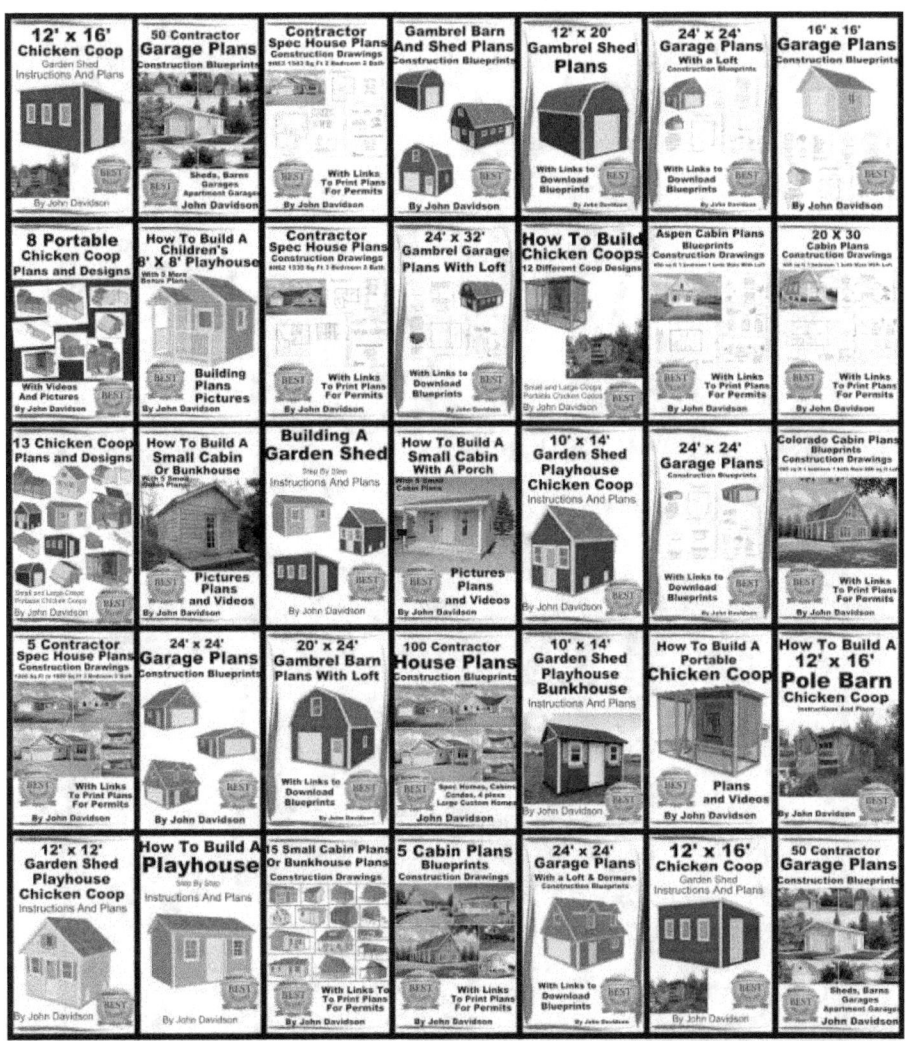

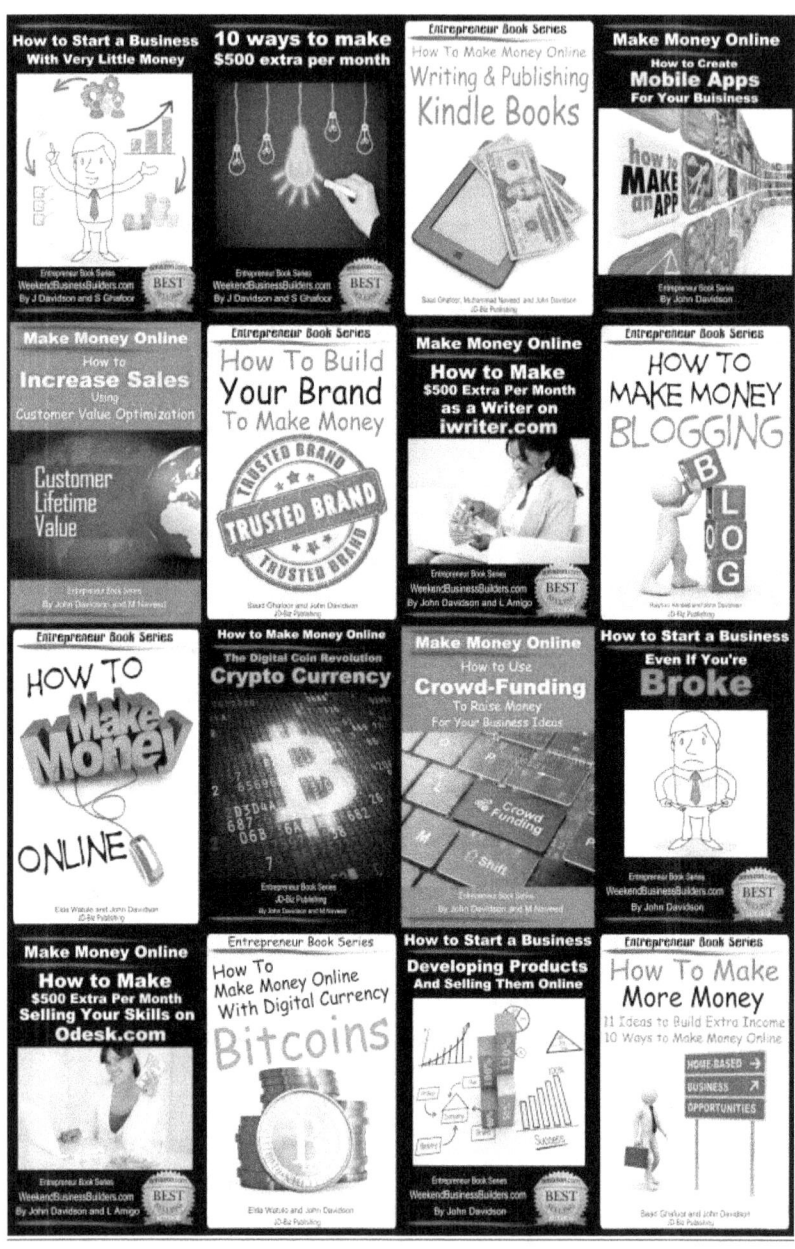

Publisher

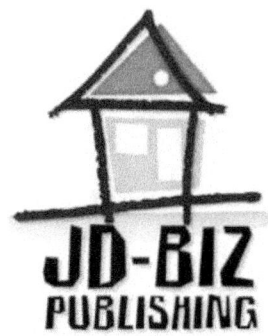

JD-Biz Corp

P O Box 374

Mendon, Utah 84325

http://www.jd-biz.com/

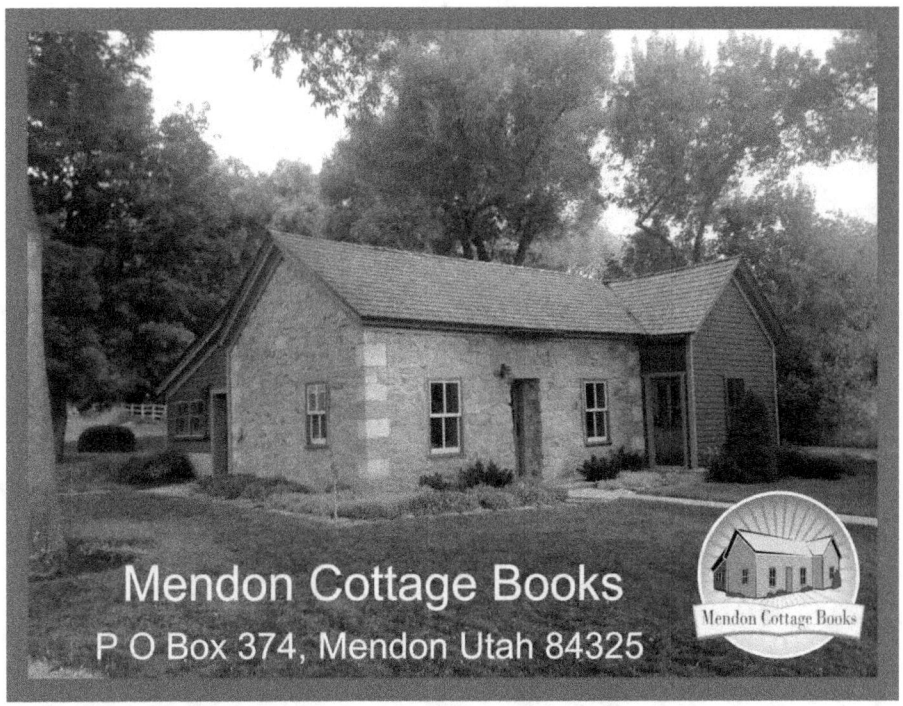

Mendon Cottage Books

P O Box 374, Mendon Utah 84325